CLEFT LIP SURGERY DIET

Unlocking The Power Of Nutrition And Empowering Wellness For Lip Surgery Healing

DR LUCAS KAYCE

DISCLAIMER

This book about illness and nutrition is not meant to replace expert medical advice, diagnosis, or treatment; rather, it is meant purely for informational reasons. This book's content is founded on broad concepts and recommendations for managing diseases and nutrition.

Before adopting any major dietary or lifestyle changes, readers are recommended to speak with a qualified healthcare provider, such as a licensed physician or registered dietitian, especially if they have pre-existing medical concerns. Everybody has different health demands, so what works for one person might not work for another.

The use of the information provided in this book may have unfavorable repercussions or consequences, for which the author and publisher disclaim all liability. No disease is meant to be identified, treated, cured, or prevented by the information provided.

The book may include contain references to medical literature or research findings; however readers are urged to independently confirm this material and contact reliable sources.

It is important to remember that the fields of nutrition and medicine are always changing, and that new findings could have an impact on the advice offered in this book. As a result, readers are urged to keep up with the most recent advancements in healthcare and, when in doubt, seek professional counsel.

By reading this book, readers agree that they are in charge of their own health decisions and release the author and publisher from any liability arising from the use of the material in the book, whether direct or indirect.

TABLE OF CONTENTS

CHAPTER ONE 11

  CLEFT LIP SURGERY DIET OVERVIEW....................................11

    KNOWLEDGE OF CLEFT LIP AND PALATE.....................11

    TYPES AND DEFINITIONS..11

    REASONS AND DANGER FACTORS.................................12

    DIET IS IMPORTANT FOR RECOVERY AFTER CLEFT LIP SURGERY 12

CHAPTER TWO 15

  IN ADVANCE OF CLEFT LIP SURGERY.................................15

    AN OVERVIEW OF SURGERY FOR CLEFT LIP 15

    DIETARY GUIDELINES BEFORE SURGERY 15

    DIETARY NEEDS 16

    FOODS TO TAKE AND LEAVE OUT 16

CHAPTER THREE 19

  DIET IMMEDIATELY FOLLOWING SURGERY.....................19

    AN OVERVIEW OF THE POSTOPERATIVE DIET.............19

    THE CLEAR LIQUID DIET...19

    CHANGE TO A COMPLETELY LIQUID DIET: 20

    THE VALUE OF HYDRATION 21

CHAPTER FOUR 23

  THE PHASE OF THE SOFT DIET 23

    SLOWLY INTRODUCING SOFT FOODS...........................23

    RICH IN NUTRIENTS CHOICES 24

    ADVICE FOR SIMPLE CONSUMPTION 24

CHAPTER FIVE...27

FULFILLING NUTRITIOUS REQUIREMENTS 27

   VITAL ELEMENTS FOR HEALING 27

   MAKING WELL-COMPOSED MEALS.......................................28

   SUPPLEMENTS FOR NUTRITION 29

CHAPTER SIX...31

   MEAL PLANS AND RECIPES..31

   RICH IN NUTRIENT RECIPES...31

   EXAMPLE MENUS FOR DIFFERENT REHAB STAGES 32

CHAPTER SEVEN 35

   LONG-TERM NUTRITIONAL CONSIDERATIONS.....................35

   POST-SURGERY NUTRITION FOR DEVELOPMENT AND GROWTH 35

   PARTICULAR FOOD RECOMMENDATIONS FOR KIDS AND TEENS 36

   LIFESTYLE AND NUTRITIONAL DECISIONS 37

CHAPTER EIGHT..39

   TAKING CARE OF ISSUES AND CHALLENGES 39

   CHEWING AND SWALLOWING DIFFICULTIES 39

   TAKING CARE OF FOOD AVERSIONS...................................39

   MEETING WITH A NUTRITIONIST 40

CHAPTER NINE 43

   EMOTIONAL ASSISTANCE AND WELFARE............................43

   PSYCHOSOCIAL ASPECTS OF RECUPERATION FROM CLEFT LIP SURGERY 43

   SUPPORT SYSTEMS FOR PATIENTS AND FAMILIES.............44

   SELF-CARE STRATEGIES 46

ABOUT THE BOOK

The "Cleft Lip Surgery Diet" book is an invaluable resource for detailed advice on the nutritional aspects of recovering from cleft lip surgery. Comprehending the complexities of cleft lip and palate is essential to realizing the importance of a customized diet for patients following surgery. The definition, kinds, causes, and risk factors of cleft lip are covered in detail in the first few chapters, which also lay the groundwork for a thorough examination of the role nutrition plays in the healing process.

The book walks readers through each stage of the recovery process after cleft lip surgery, beginning with the preoperative planning and ending with the first postoperative phase. It carefully describes what foods to include or avoid, as well as nutritional needs and preoperative dietary instructions. This methodical approach guarantees that readers understand the critical actions to follow to maximize recovery results before surgery.

The initial postoperative period is given special attention, with ideas like clear liquid and entire liquid diets introduced. Emphasis is placed on the significance of staying hydrated, acknowledging its critical function in the healing process.

The shift to a soft diet is covered in later chapters, along with helpful hints on how to include nutrient-dense soft foods in the postoperative diet. This sequence of events corresponds with the changing nutritional requirements of those pursuing recuperation.

The book delves deeper into the long-term aspects of post-operative nutrition, emphasizing the vital nutrients needed for long-term healing and development. It acknowledges the difficulties people could experience, like trouble swallowing and chewing, and offers workable answers. Furthermore, the incorporation of recipes and meal planning guarantees that readers possess concrete resources to proficiently execute the dietary guidelines.

Interestingly, the book addresses the psychosocial components of healing in addition to the physical ones. A section on emotional support and well-being is devoted to it, recognizing the significance of a comprehensive approach to the healing process. Through the inclusion of lifestyle factors, nutritional recommendations, and support networks, the book provides a thorough resource for patients, families, and medical professionals involved in the healing process following cleft lip surgery.

"Cleft Lip Surgery Diet" proves to be a useful manual that blends medical knowledge with useful guidance, providing a comprehensive strategy for nutritional support throughout the healing process. With its thorough examination of every stage, as well as its recipes, meal plans, and techniques for providing emotional support, the book establishes itself as a valuable tool for anybody navigating the challenges of recovering from cleft lip surgery.

CHAPTER ONE

KNOWLEDGE OF CLEFT LIP AND PALATE

Congenital disorders that alter a person's facial anatomy, such as cleft lip and palate, offer particular difficulties and call for specific medical attention. These disorders cause holes or clefts in the upper lip and/or palate due to insufficient fusion of the face tissues during embryonic development. Healthcare professionals, patients, and their families must manage the complexity of diagnosis, treatment, and rehabilitation by having a thorough understanding of the nuances of cleft lip and palate.

TYPES AND DEFINITIONS

Orofacial clefts, which include cleft lip and palate, are a group of disorders that differ in severity and appearance. A cleft lip is a separation or gap in the upper lip. It can vary in size from a tiny notch to a larger split that reaches into the nose.

A cleft palate, on the other hand, affects either the soft or hard palate and is caused by a gap in the roof of the mouth. Cleft lip and palate can be the outcome of either ailment alone or in combination.

REASONS AND DANGER FACTORS

Cleft lip and palate have a complex etiology that involves both hereditary and environmental variables. Environmental variables are important, but genetic predisposition is also present, with a higher risk for those with a family history of orofacial clefts. Cleft lip and palate have been associated with maternal exposure to teratogenic drugs such as alcohol, tobacco smoke, and certain medications during pregnancy. Furthermore, poor nutrition and older mothers are seen as possible risk factors.

DIET IS IMPORTANT FOR RECOVERY AFTER CLEFT LIP SURGERY

Following cleft lip surgery, diet is highly important because proper healing and general health depend on nutritional assistance. People who have had cleft lip surgery could have trouble feeding; therefore they would need to adjust their diet to make sure they are getting enough food.

For infants with cleft lip, specialist feeding methods including using nipples and specialty bottles may be advised to help with optimal nutrition.

In addition, easy-to-eat foods that don't put too much strain on the healing surgical site are part of the postoperative dietary concerns. Sufficient hydration and a nutritious, well-balanced diet are vital elements of the healing process that promote tissue repair and reduce the likelihood of problems.

To effectively manage the difficulties posed by these congenital disorders, healthcare professionals, patients, and their families must have a thorough awareness of the complexity surrounding cleft lip and palate. This introduction offers a thorough review of the complexities of cleft lip and palate, covering everything from describing the numerous forms of orofacial clefts to investigating the complex causes and risk factors. Furthermore, stressing the role nutrition plays during the recuperation stage emphasizes the necessity for a comprehensive strategy to meet the specific requirements of patients after cleft lip surgery.

CHAPTER TWO

IN ADVANCE OF CLEFT LIP SURGERY

AN OVERVIEW OF SURGERY FOR CLEFT LIP

The goal of reconstructive surgery for cleft lip is to close an opening or gap in the upper lip caused by a congenital defect. This disorder develops when the tissues that make up the upper lip fail to fuse entirely during fetal development. Early infancy is the usual time for cleft lip surgery to treat the condition's functional and cosmetic components. The ultimate objective is to return the lip to its natural structure, which will enhance face symmetry, speaking, and general well-being.

DIETARY GUIDELINES BEFORE SURGERY

Preoperative food instructions should be carefully considered before having cleft lip surgery to maintain good health and facilitate a speedy recovery. The body needs proper nutrition to help tissue repair, strengthen the immune system, and get ready for surgery.

Patients who are going to get cleft lip surgery should follow a diet that is well-balanced and rich in different nutrients.

DIETARY NEEDS

Before cleft lip surgery, the diet must include essential components such as protein, vitamins, and minerals. Protein is necessary for wound healing and for repairing damaged tissue. Thus, people should incorporate foods high in protein in their diets, such as fish, eggs, dairy products, lean meats, and plant-based foods like tofu and lentils. Enough consumption of vitamins and minerals is essential for immune system support and appropriate healing, particularly for zinc, vitamin C, and vitamin A.

FOODS TO TAKE AND LEAVE OUT

Nutrient-dense and readily digested foods should be a part of the preoperative diet. The following should be given priority: lean proteins, fruits, vegetables, and whole grains.

A variety of vitamins and minerals found in these foods support general health and aid in the body's preparation for surgery. Furthermore important is hydration; people should drink enough water to avoid becoming dehydrated, which might impede the healing process.

However, some foods should be avoided before cleft lip surgery. Sugary and highly processed meals should be consumed in moderation since they may weaken the immune system and cause inflammation.

To further reduce pain before and after surgery, foods that are hard to chew or could irritate the digestive tract should be avoided. It is essential to speak with a nutritionist or healthcare provider to develop a customized preoperative meal plan based on the patient's unique requirements and medical background.

Cleft lip surgery preparation entails a comprehensive approach that considers the patient's general health as well as the surgical technique. Strict adherence to preoperative dietary recommendations, an emphasis on nutritional needs, and awareness of what foods to eat and avoid can all help ensure a successful surgical procedure and a more seamless recuperation. To maximize the results of cleft lip surgery, patients must collaborate closely with their healthcare team to make sure that their dietary demands are satisfied.

CHAPTER THREE

DIET IMMEDIATELY FOLLOWING SURGERY

AN OVERVIEW OF THE POSTOPERATIVE DIET

For people who have had surgery, the postoperative phase is crucial to their recuperation. To assist the body's healing processes and rebuild strength following surgery, proper nutrition is essential. The patient's initial postoperative diet is specially designed to satisfy their nutritional demands while taking into account their tolerance for and capacity to digest various types of food. Before introducing more solid foods, the shift from fasting to oral intake usually entails a slow development through several diet phases, beginning with a clear liquid diet and progressing to a full liquid diet.

THE CLEAR LIQUID DIET

The first phase in the postoperative nutritional progression is frequently the clear liquid diet.

The ingestion of clear, easily digested fluids is part of this phase. Clear liquids include things like broth, water, gelatin, and clear juices. This diet gives the body the vital fluids it needs to stay hydrated, especially in cases where patients may still be recuperating from anesthesia. Clear drinks are a good option for the initial phases of postoperative recovery since they leave less residue behind and are less prone to aggravate the digestive tract. During this stage, medical professionals can keep an eye on the patient's oral intake tolerance and determine whether they're ready to move on to the following nutritional stage.

CHANGE TO A COMPLETELY LIQUID DIET:

Patients usually move on to a full liquid diet after completing the clear liquid phase. More variety and nutritional content are introduced at this time, along with pureed foods, milk-based products, and smooth soups. Full liquids are a good option for people who may still feel some discomfort or have trouble swallowing after surgery because they are simpler to swallow and digest than solid foods. The complete liquid diet supplies the vital minerals, proteins, and calories the body needs for energy needs and the healing process. Healthcare practitioners can further tailor the diet plan to each patient's unique nutritional requirements when they show signs of increased tolerance and gastrointestinal function.

THE VALUE OF HYDRATION

A crucial component of the postoperative diet and the healing process is staying hydrated. Sustaining electrolyte balance, avoiding dehydration, and promoting general physiological processes all depend on adequate fluid intake.

Patients may lose more fluids in the early postoperative phase for a variety of reasons, including medication side effects, restricted oral intake, and stress after the surgery. Maintaining adequate hydration is essential for accelerating the healing of wounds, averting complications, and enhancing organ performance.

Healthcare professionals keep a careful eye on their patients' fluid status and modify their hydration regimens as necessary. Maintaining adequate fluid balance is essential to the success of the entire postoperative care plan, and stressing the importance of hydration during the postoperative period helps guarantee that patients are actively engaging in their recovery.

CHAPTER FOUR

THE PHASE OF THE SOFT DIET

SLOWLY INTRODUCING SOFT FOODS

One of the most important ways to facilitate a seamless shift from a liquid or pureed diet to a more varied and textured eating plan is to gradually introduce soft foods during the soft diet phase. This stage is usually advised for those who are recovering from surgeries or other medical treatments, or who have trouble swallowing or chewing. Soft foods should be added gradually to assist the digestive system adjust while reducing discomfort and guaranteeing enough nourishment.

Introducing soft foods is adding foods that are simple to chew and swallow, like soft fruits, tender meats, and well-cooked vegetables. By taking it slowly, the person may acclimate to the different textures and reacquaint their jaw muscles with chewing motions.

Before moving on to more complicated textures, it can be a moderate approach to start the soft diet phase with foods that are readily digested, such as pureed soups or mashed potatoes.

RICH IN NUTRIENTS CHOICES

During the soft diet phase, nutrient-rich alternatives are essential for sustaining good health. While softer textures are the major focus, it's crucial to make sure the diet still offers the necessary nutrients and is well-balanced.

Eating foods high in protein, such as yogurt, eggs, and finely ground meats, supports the body's ability to repair muscles and operate as a whole. Incorporating nutrient-dense foods like avocados, soft-cooked beans, and fortified cereals into a well-rounded diet also helps to ward off certain nutrient deficits.

ADVICE FOR SIMPLE CONSUMPTION

Suggestions for convenient eating throughout the soft diet stage can improve people's experiences in general during this phase of change.

Even with soft foods, chewing slowly and thoroughly encourages healthy digestion and lowers the possibility of discomfort. Managing appetite and avoiding jaw muscle overuse can also be aided by dividing meals into smaller, more frequent amounts throughout the day.

Trying out various cooking methods, such as steaming or slow cooking, will help soften food without sacrificing its nutritious value, which will make it simpler to eat and more pleasant.

Apart from choosing soft foods, some goods can be made easier to consume by changing their texture. For example, pureeing veggies into soups or blending fruits into smoothies can be an easy method to add vital nutrients with a smoother consistency. It is important to consider personal preferences and to progressively reintroduce different textures as the person becomes used to chewing and swallowing them.

The soft diet phase is a transitional phase that calls for a careful strategy to guarantee comfort and adequate nourishment.

A successful and fulfilling experience during this phase is largely dependent on the gradual introduction of soft foods, the inclusion of nutrient-rich options, and the adoption of suggestions for simple ingestion, all of which eventually promote the individual's general well-being.

CHAPTER FIVE

FULFILLING NUTRITIOUS REQUIREMENTS

VITAL ELEMENTS FOR HEALING

Fulfilling nutritional requirements is essential for general health and well-being, especially for recuperating after physical strain, disease, or trauma. The body's regeneration and repair processes depend heavily on essential nutrients. Of them, protein is particularly important as a building block for healing. Protein is vital for muscle recovery since it is necessary for tissue development and repair. Lean meats, dairy products, legumes, and nuts are among the foods that supply the essential amino acids required for tissue repair and healing.

Apart from protein, vitamins and minerals play an equally important role in the healing process. Vitamins, like vitamin C, are essential for the creation of collagen, which promotes tissue and wound healing.

Certain minerals, such as magnesium and zinc, are necessary for both muscular contractions and immune system operation, which aids in the process of healing. A diet rich in a range of fruits, vegetables, and whole grains guarantees a sufficient intake of essential micronutrients, which aid in the body's healing processes.

MAKING WELL-COMPOSED MEALS

For satiating dietary requirements and maintaining energy levels throughout the day, balanced meals are crucial. A balanced meal usually consists of a range of micronutrients from fruits and vegetables as well as macronutrients like proteins, fats, and carbs. The main source of energy is found in carbohydrates, proteins aid in the maintenance and repair of muscles, and fats aid in satiety and the absorption of fat-soluble vitamins.

Meals containing complex carbs, including whole grains, are essential for recovery because they restore glycogen stores and give long-lasting energy.

Lean protein foods including fish, poultry, tofu, and beans guarantee a sufficient amount of amino acids for muscle repair. Nuts, avocados, and olive oil are good sources of healthy fats that promote nutrient absorption and general well-being. To ensure that the body gets a wide range of nutrients necessary for healing, creating balanced meals demands paying attention to portion sizes and a diversity of food types.

SUPPLEMENTS FOR NUTRITION

Although the best source of nutrients should be whole foods, there are situations when taking nutritional supplements can help fill up any gaps in a person's diet. Supplements can help athletes, people on a restricted diet, and people recuperating from illnesses fulfill their higher nutritional needs. Whey and plant-based powder supplements are two easy ways to increase protein consumption for muscle repair.

Supplements containing vitamins and minerals may be advised when food consumption is inadequate or during times of high demand, such as rigorous training or the healing process following surgery. However, it's important to use supplements sparingly because taking too many of them can cause imbalances and even pose health hazards. The proper usage of supplements can be determined by speaking with a trained nutritionist or healthcare expert, depending on the needs and circumstances of each individual.

Addressing nutritional requirements for healing necessitates a comprehensive strategy that includes a diet that is well-balanced and full of vital nutrients. The body's healing processes depend heavily on protein, vitamins, and minerals, and eating balanced meals guarantees a varied and complete diet. In certain circumstances, nutritional supplements can be beneficial additions, but to minimize hazards, they should only be used sparingly and under the supervision of a professional.

CHAPTER SIX

MEAL PLANS AND RECIPES

RICH IN NUTRIENT RECIPES

Recipes that are high in nutrients are vital for maintaining general health and well-being because they supply the vitamins, minerals, and other nutrients that the body needs to perform at its best. By using a variety of nutrient-dense products, these dishes are made to maximize nutritious content. These recipes frequently have an emphasis on a well-balanced mix of healthy fats, proteins, carbs, vitamins, and minerals to make sure that people are getting a wide variety of nutrients at every meal.

When it comes to nutrient-dense dishes, whole, unprocessed ingredients are frequently the main focus. Lean proteins that are high in critical amino acids for muscle growth and repair include fish, fowl, tofu, and lentils. Complex carbs are provided by whole grains like quinoa, brown rice, and oats, while a range of vibrant fruits and vegetables offer a wealth of vitamins, minerals, and antioxidants. The addition of healthy fats from nuts, avocados, and olive oil helps to enhance nutritional absorption and brain health.

Nutrient-dense dishes can also be adjusted to accommodate different dietary needs and constraints. Whatever one's dietary restrictions—vegetarian, vegan, gluten-free, or otherwise—the focus always needs to be on producing tasty, nutrient-dense meals. Improving general health as well as supporting particular health goals like better digestion, weight control, or increased athletic performance are the main aims.

EXAMPLE MENUS FOR DIFFERENT REHAB STAGES

Designed to meet individual health demands, sample meal plans for different stages of recovery make sure people eat enough throughout times of healing or rehabilitation. To support tissue healing and immunological function, easily digestible foods high in protein could be the main focus of post-surgery recovery meal programs. These menus may consist of soups, lean meats, and nutrient-dense smoothies.

On the other hand, meal plans for athletes in the recuperation stage can place more emphasis on the timing of nutrients to maximize muscle repair and glycogen resupply.

It is essential to include a balance of proteins and carbohydrates as well as hydration choices to aid with their recuperation. Meal plans for people with chronic illnesses or in recovery may be created to manage dietary limitations or specific nutritional shortages while fostering general health.

Meal plans can also be modified to take into account aspects of lifestyle like dietary restrictions or hectic schedules. For people who don't have much time to prepare meals, quick and simple nutrient-dense recipes can be added, guaranteeing that convenience doesn't sacrifice nutritious value. Additionally, a range of tastes and culinary traditions can be included to create meal plans that are sustainable and pleasurable for people in various stages of recovery.

Healthy recipes and sample meal plans are essential parts of an all-encompassing strategy for wellness and recuperation. From post-surgery rehabilitation to sports recuperation and beyond, these approaches promote different stages of recovery and enhance general well-being by emphasizing full, nutrient-dense meals and customizing meal plans to meet individual needs.

CHAPTER SEVEN

LONG-TERM NUTRITIONAL CONSIDERATIONS

POST-SURGERY NUTRITION FOR DEVELOPMENT AND GROWTH

Nutrition following surgery is essential for promoting development and growth, particularly in kids and teenagers. The metabolism, nutritional condition, and absorption of nutrients can all be affected by surgical treatments. Following surgery, the healing process may increase the body's need for energy and nutrients. It becomes essential to customize the food to support the best possible recovery and long-term growth.

Protein is essential for post-surgery nutrition because it supports immunological and tissue healing. Consuming enough protein promotes muscle growth and the healing of surgical wounds. Additionally, consuming foods high in antioxidants, zinc, and vitamin C is crucial for boosting immunity and lowering the chance of infection while recovering.

After surgery, calorie requirements could go up to accommodate the higher energy requirements linked to the healing process. To avoid excessive weight gain, which could impede healing; it is crucial to find a balance. Developing a customized post-surgical nutrition plan that takes into consideration the patient's age, weight, and type of surgery is a critical task that requires collaboration with healthcare specialists, including nutritionists and surgeons.

PARTICULAR FOOD RECOMMENDATIONS FOR KIDS AND TEENS

The fast growth and development of children and adolescents means that they have special nutritional needs. To address these factors, a thorough grasp of their nutritional needs at various life stages is necessary. In addition to being essential for physical growth, a healthy diet also affects immunological response, cognitive development, and general well-being.

Focusing on nutrient-dense meals during childhood is critical because they offer the vitamins and minerals required for optimal bone development, cognitive function, and the formation of good eating habits. It is especially important to consume enough calcium and vitamin D to maintain bone health and avoid problems like osteoporosis later in life.

Adolescence presents a unique set of difficulties, such as elevated energy requirements and the possibility of unhealthful eating patterns. It is crucial to promote a varied, well-balanced diet full of fruits, vegetables, healthy grains, and lean meats. Adolescents' general well-being is also enhanced by addressing issues with body image, encouraging a positive connection with food, and teaching them how to make smart eating choices.

LIFESTYLE AND NUTRITIONAL DECISIONS

An essential component of long-term health is the confluence of food decisions and lifestyle choices. To enhance general well-being, lifestyle elements like exercise, stress reduction, and enough sleep are just as important as food selections.

Frequent exercise enhances cardiovascular health, muscular strength, and mental well-being in addition to helping with weight management.

Comprehending the significance of a well-rounded and diverse diet is vital for making knowledgeable dietary decisions. Including a diverse array of nutrients from several food categories guarantees that the body gets the vital vitamins, minerals, and macronutrients required for optimum performance. It is imperative to abstain from bad fats, added sugars, and processed meals to prevent chronic diseases including obesity, diabetes, and cardiovascular problems.

Maintaining long-term dietary changes also requires careful consideration of cultural and personal preferences. Healthy eating habits are encouraged when a flexible strategy that allows for a variety of food choices while preserving nutritional balance is used. A sustainable and health-promoting way of life is built on the synergy between dietary choices and lifestyle choices with the goal of long-term well-being.

CHAPTER EIGHT

TAKING CARE OF ISSUES AND CHALLENGES

CHEWING AND SWALLOWING DIFFICULTIES

Promoting general health and well-being requires addressing issues with eating habits. One typical dietary obstacle that people may experience is swallowing and chewing difficulties. Numerous variables, including dental abnormalities, jaw issues, or neurological conditions, may give rise to this problem. It is imperative to employ a customized approach that considers the root cause to address this challenge. For example, people with dental problems might benefit from dental procedures, but people with neurological impairments might need specialist therapies to enhance their ability to swallow and chew food.

TAKING CARE OF FOOD AVERSIONS

Another major obstacle to keeping a balanced diet is food aversions. Aversions to particular foods can arise for several reasons, such as sensory problems, unpleasant experiences in the past, or cultural influences. To address food aversions, a supportive environment that motivates people to try new foods must be established.

A more varied and nutrient-dense diet can be promoted and preferences can be reshaped with the help of gradual exposure and positive reinforcement. Involving a nutritionist or mental health professional in the process can also yield insightful advice and helpful coping mechanisms for aversions.

MEETING WITH A NUTRITIONIST

A proactive approach to addressing and managing nutritional issues is consulting with a dietician. Dietitians are qualified experts who can evaluate a person's nutritional requirements, take into account particular medical issues, and offer individualized dietary advice. People can learn a lot about managing dietary restrictions, choosing healthy foods, and attaining overall nutritional balance by working with a nutritionist. Together, with consideration for each person's lifestyle, tastes, and health objectives, this collaborative method guarantees that dietary programs are not only sustainable but also beneficial.

When a person has trouble chewing and swallowing, a dietitian can create customized meal plans that meet their unique requirements. To guarantee sufficient nutritional intake, this may entail suggesting foods with softer textures, pureed foods, or liquid supplements.

A dietitian can help people with food aversions by introducing nutrient-rich, alternative options that are tailored to the individual's taste preferences, thereby diversifying their diet. The dietitian can also provide advice on behavioral techniques to gradually overcome aversions and mindful eating habits.

Furthermore, talking with a dietitian covers long-term dietary management in addition to immediate problems. To maintain a positive relationship with food, dietitians can help with goal-setting, habit creation, and continuous support. This cooperative method recognizes each person's particular situation and gives them the ability to make knowledgeable food decisions that will improve their general health and way of life.

CHAPTER NINE

EMOTIONAL ASSISTANCE AND WELFARE

PSYCHOSOCIAL ASPECTS OF RECUPERATION FROM CLEFT LIP SURGERY

Recovery from cleft lip surgery requires careful attention to important psychosocial factors in addition to physical healing. After undergoing this procedure, patients may feel a variety of emotions, such as anxiety, altered self-esteem, and self-consciousness. Because cleft lip conditions are visible, feelings of social stigmatization may arise, which may hurt an individual's mental health. For a complete recovery, these psychosocial factors must be addressed.

Notable is the effect of cleft lip surgery on one's perception of oneself. Patients may struggle with worries about how they look and what other people think of them. Increased self-awareness and, in certain situations, difficulties forming and sustaining relationships can result from this. Individuals need psychosocial support, such as peer relationships and counseling, to effectively manage these emotional obstacles.

Moreover, family dynamics are affected psychologically. While they assist their child in recovering, parents and other caregivers may go through emotional turmoil. Coping with the visible effects of surgery and managing societal attitudes toward their child's condition can be emotionally taxing. Integrating psychological support into the overall care plan is essential to address the emotional well-being of both the patient and their family.

SUPPORT SYSTEMS FOR PATIENTS AND FAMILIES

Creating a robust support system is paramount for patients and their families during the cleft lip surgery recovery journey. Peer support groups and counseling services can offer a platform for individuals to share their experiences, providing mutual understanding and encouragement.

Connecting with others who have undergone similar challenges fosters a sense of community and reduces feelings of isolation.

Medical professionals, including surgeons, nurses, and psychologists, are integral components of the support system. These experts play a crucial role in providing information, addressing concerns, and guiding patients and their families through the recovery process. Establishing open lines of communication between healthcare providers and families helps build trust and ensures that emotional and informational needs are met.

Educational resources are valuable tools for patients and families to gain a better understanding of cleft lip conditions and the associated surgical procedures. Access to accurate information empowers individuals to make informed decisions and promotes a sense of control over their situation. Support organizations and online forums can serve as additional resources, offering a wealth of information and fostering a sense of belonging.

SELF-CARE STRATEGIES

Self-care is a fundamental aspect of emotional well-being during the recovery from cleft lip surgery. Patients and their families should prioritize activities that promote relaxation, reduce stress, and enhance overall mental health. Engaging in hobbies, practicing mindfulness techniques, and maintaining a healthy lifestyle contribute to a positive mindset.

Open communication within the family is essential for emotional support. Encouraging an environment where feelings and concerns can be openly expressed helps build resilience and strengthens familial bonds. Setting realistic expectations and celebrating small victories in the recovery process can contribute to a positive outlook and enhance the overall well-being of the patient.

Additionally, seeking professional counseling or therapy is a proactive self-care strategy.

Mental health professionals can provide tools to cope with emotional challenges, facilitate communication within the family, and address any lingering psychological effects of the surgery. Prioritizing mental and emotional health is crucial for a comprehensive and successful recovery from cleft lip surgery.

9 798888 029076 5